Choose Your Words

Melanie Sears, R.N., M.B.A., Ph.D.

Harnessing the Power of Compassionate
Communication to Heal and Connect

www.dnadialogues.com

CREDITS
Production and Content Coordinator: Sara Saltee of Strategic Learning Resources, Inc.
Images: Dreamstime.com
Design: Soundview Design Studio

Contents

Activity Guide

REFLECTION TOPICS

EXERCISES

Overview
& Highlights

OVERVIEW

Communicating with a client who has been diagnosed with a mental illness can be frustrating and emotionally draining. Being in a position of "the authority" can create walls between you and the other person and will prevent authentic connection and growth from occurring. This guidebook offers a system called Nonviolent Communication that will give you specific tools you can use to support your clients, point them in the direction of health and balance, and maintain honest, open dialogues. You will learn how to transform negative patterns and bridge the gap that separates you from your clients, find out what words are likely to trigger defensive reactions from them, and discover what you can say that will create safety and open-hearted communication. The guidebook demonstrates how to be compassionate to others even when you don't agree with their point of view and will offer ways you can care for yourself in the midst of the challenges you are facing.

HIGHLIGHTS

In this guidebook, you will learn:

◆ What the habitual patterns of communication are.

◆ How Nonviolent Communication can transform interactions.

◆ The four steps of Nonviolent Communication.

◆ How to express empathy for self.

◆ Ways to express empathy to others.

You will Practice:

◆ Observing your habitual communication patterns.

◆ Expressing your honesty using the model of Nonviolent Communication.

◆ Separating observation from evaluation.

◆ Expressing feelings in a self-responsible manner.

◆ Clearly stating your needs.

◆ Making clear requests.

◆ Translating judgments into feelings and needs.

◆ Giving empathy to someone who is distressed.

◆ Taking care of your own needs.

◆ Giving yourself empathy when you are distressed.

◆ Translating your inner judgments into feelings and needs.

You will take away:

- ♦ A set of powerful and effective tools to use in all your inter-actions with others.

- ♦ A guide for self-responsibility and self-empowerment.

- ♦ Understanding of communication dynamics.

- ♦ Understanding of how to express compassion even in trying circumstances.

- ♦ Knowledge of how to care for your own needs in spite of outward demands.

- ♦ A model for creating caring connections and understanding between you and your clients.

CHAPTER 1

Introduction

SANDY'S STORY

Sandy had been seeing Bill, a thirty-two-year-old patient who was diagnosed with paranoid schizophrenia, for four months. She felt frustrated that she could not connect with him and annoyed to see him make the same self-destructive choices time after time. Sandy doubted that she could do anything to help him. She saw him as a hopeless case with a chronic mental illness. She felt angry when he cussed her out and criticized her efforts to help. Sandy tried setting limits by telling him, "I'm going to have to end this session if you continue treating me in a disrespectful way." He continued to swear at her. Their interactions were becoming so painful that she didn't want to be his clinician any more.

Many clinicians find it difficult to communicate with clients who are severely ill. How do you know how to say the right thing, or at least how not to say the wrong thing? How can you keep a sense of connection to someone who judges and blames you? Like Sandy, you may find yourself walking on eggshells, not sure how to bridge the gap between you and the one you wish to help. You have found that using power over techniques alienates your client, but how do you protect yourself if you don't play the *authority* card?

Knowing what to say that will open up communication and create harmonious connections is indeed a challenge. This guidebook will help you meet that challenge by introducing you to specific tools you can use to communicate in ways that move you toward – not away from – those you work with, even when they are at their most difficult. You'll have many opportunities along the way to practice with these new tools, and you'll follow Sandy's progress, too, as she uses them to transform her awareness and her communication and begins to change the confusing interactions she has with Bill.

WHAT IS NONVIOLENT COMMUNICATION?

Nonviolent Communication was created about forty-five years ago by Dr. Marshall Rosenberg. As he studied the question, "What keeps us connected to our naturally compassionate nature?" he discovered the importance of how we use words. He studied people who were considered "good" communicators and broke down what they were doing into four steps. From these steps, he developed the model of Nonviolent Communication that he teaches today. Indeed, Dr. Rosenberg travels all over the world teaching this process, resolving conflicts in war-torn countries, and helping people live peaceful, joyful lives by shifting their communication.

Nonviolent Communication creates peaceful connections between people, regardless of whom the tools are used with. Using NVC is more challenging with the people we are closest with because those patterns of communication are emotionally charged, but learning to use these tools can be a healing process for everyone involved. The NVC tools are effective in all kinds of different situations, from your most intimate relationships, to your professional life, to your interactions with doctors and others on your care team. These tools work well in mediation, in conflict resolution, and in creating soul-satisfying intimacy. NVC is even effective when you are the only one using it.

The core premise of Nonviolent Communication is that our pattern of internal and external communication creates the world we experience. When we become conscious of our communication and develop choice in how we think and react, then we change our world. In this way, Nonviolent Communication shifts our relationship to our world and enables us to create worlds that expand rather than limit possibility for ourselves and those around us.

This guidebook walks you through the principles of Nonviolent Communication and helps you apply them to the specific situations you find yourself in as someone who works with and cares about a person who has mental illness. We'll look at ways to stay connected to others and yourself even when you are dealing with difficult dynamics, such as when someone cusses at you, or when someone refuses to speak at all, or when someone communicates about a delusional world.

The guidebook will first clarify communication patterns that are not helpful in creating a safe connection with others. Then the process of Nonviolent Communication will unfold. You will learn how to express your truth in a way that is least likely to trigger a defensive reaction in others. Then you will learn how to clearly hear what is in the heart of another person, even if that person is judging and blaming you. You will learn how to not take things personally. Finally you will understand what is behind your own judgments and learn to treat yourself in a compassionate manner.

The information in this guidebook can shift frustrating dynamics between you and your clients and create accelerated growth for your clients. My guess is that these tools will not only be useful for you as a clinician, they will be useful in helping you navigate through all the interactions in your life. You will learn how to create deeper levels of intimacy in your relationships, begin to hear others very differently, and develop skills that can help heal the emotional wounds that prevent you from getting what you need.

PERSONAL ⊘ REFLECTION

REFLECTION TOPIC 1: A COMMUNICATION CHALLENGE

By way of introduction to the material in this guidebook, think about a communication challenge with a client you are facing today. What is the communication dynamic you'd most like to change?

CHAPTER 2

Breaking Old Habits

CHANGE YOUR WORDS, CHANGE YOUR RELATIONSHIPS

Many of us communicate in ways we hardly notice, relying on habits and patterns we developed in childhood. Quite often, these unconsidered communication habits keep us stuck in painful relationship dynamics with those we care about the most.

The purpose of NVC is to introduce some new communication patterns, patterns that create connections and help people get their deepest needs met. To create this type of connection, we need to unlearn some of our destructive communication patterns and learn ways of communicating that create a kind of safe space within which honesty can be expressed.

You'll find a strong focus on language in this guidebook, with lots of close-up looks at the specific words you may habitually use and words that can do a better job for you.

> Language both creates and expresses consciousness.

The reason for this emphasis on words is that language creates and expresses consciousness, and language shapes the way that others respond to you. The words we use can trigger reactions in other people. If we use words that express judgments, labels, or other forms of prescriptive communication, we can expect defensive reactions from others. NVC teaches us that when we use words that take responsibility for our feelings and needs, people will react differently toward us.

COMMON PATTERNS OF RESPONSE

Below, you'll see a list of habits many of us fall into when we are communicating with others. Most of us draw from a range of these patterns in our conversation, but some fall into a groove of responding most frequently in one or two different ways. When you think about people in your life with whom you talk regularly, you might notice that they most frequently fall into a few of these patterns.

Do you have a colleague who always meets one of your stories with a story of how that very thing happened to her? Maybe you've met someone who always wants to teach you everything he knows about the topic at hand? And what about you? Do you see some patterns of response in this list that you think you frequently rely on?

A Short List of Habitual Responses

- Judgment
- Analysis
- Diagnosis
- Labeling
- Reassurance
- Advice
- Interrogating
- Fixing It

- Story Telling
- Educating
- One-Upping
- Consoling
- Shutting Down
- Sympathizing
- Explaining
- Correcting

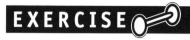

EXERCISE

EXERCISE 1: BECOMING AWARE OF COMMON COMMUNICATION PATTERNS

To develop an awareness of what these common habits of response sound like, imagine that a patient came to you and said:

"My life is a mess; I can't do anything right."

Look at the blanks below and think of responses you might offer your patient if you were speaking from the different communication patterns listed. There are no "right answers" here – just have fun with experimenting with responding in these different ways. You might gently notice, as you go, which responses come easily to you and which are more difficult. Chances are, the easy ones are the ones you personally rely on most. I've completed the first couple to get you started (turn to Page 15 to see Sandy's responses):

Judgment: "You really should have a more positive attitude."

Analysis: "The reason your life is a mess is that your parents never made you take responsibility for your actions when you were a kid."

Diagnosis

Label

Reassurance

Advice

Interrogating

Fixing It

Story Telling

Educating

One-Upping

Consoling

Shutting Down

Sympathizing

Explaining

Correcting

Remember Sandy and Bill, whom you met in the introduction? Here are some of Sandy's usual responses to Bill when he has spoken to her about his feelings of hopelessness about his life:

Judgment: *You're an emotional mess. You should be better by now.*

Analysis: *It's because you had a painful childhood.*

Diagnosis: *Because you have a diagnosis of schizophrenia, you shouldn't expect so much of yourself.*

Label: *It's because you are disabled.*

Reassurance: *Don't worry, you'll be OK.*

Advice: *Why don't you take some classes at the Community College?*

Interrogating: *How long have you felt this way?*

Fixing It: *If you took the mood stabilizer that the doctor suggested, you would feel better.*

Story Telling: *That reminds me of what another client said....*

Educating: *You'll need to take the medicine for the rest of your life.*

One Upping: *You think you feel bad? Think of all the people who can't even hold a job.*

Consoling: *It's not your fault. You do the best that you can.*

Shutting Down: *Don't worry about it. Cheer up.*

Sympathizing: *Oh, you poor thing.*

Explaining: *It's my job as your clinician to tell you what you need to do to get better.*

Correcting: *Don't think in terms of right and wrong. Think of what you can do, not what you can't.*

REFLECTION TOPIC 2:
WHAT ARE YOUR HABITS?

As you thought about possible responses and reflected on Sandy's responses, did you become more aware of your own most common communication patterns? What are they? What role you think those patterns might play in the uncomfortable communication dynamic you identified in Reflection Topic 1?

THE LANGUAGE OF BLAME

We often only learn two ways of responding to others:

1. We blame them.
2. We blame ourselves.

Either way, both responses reflect an outward focus of attention. Our attention is placed on what someone else is or what they will think of us. If we don't like what others are doing, we judge them or blame them instead of revealing what is going on inside us. For example, "If you can't understand what I said, you must be stupid," or "I don't understand what she said; she is a lousy communicator."

We can also focus our attention on labeling or blaming ourselves. Many of us have integrated labels about ourselves that we heard growing up. As we get older we use these labels to beat ourselves up with. This stimulates self-hate, which leads to depression. For example, if you are struggling to understand what someone is saying to you, you might jump to the self-accusation: "I don't understand what he means by that; I must be stupid." And we not only beat up on ourselves, we also worry about how we will be judged by others. At the same time we think, "I must be stupid," we also fear "If I reveal that I don't understand what he means by that, others will think I'm stupid." Self-judgment and fear of judgment from others are wrapped tightly together – and both cause pain.

When all our energy goes to defending ourselves from other's judgments or judging others or ourselves, the world can seem like a hostile place. This type of communication, called static language, keeps us stuck on the "hamster wheel." It does not allow us to grow and heal. It does not create loving connections, but pain and confusion.

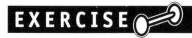
EXERCISE 2: CHECK YOUR INNER LANGUAGE

To begin this exercise, think of the last time you made a mistake. Jot your memory down on a piece of paper and write down what you did.

Now think about what you said to yourself about that mistake. What were the words running through your head after the mistake was made? Don't judge the words, just see if you can capture what you heard in your mind. Write them down.

Now, look back at what you wrote. Did it contain any of the static language patterns discussed above? Go back and underline statements that you now think might be judging, blaming, labeling, or defending.

A FOUR-STEP PROCESS

Nonviolent Communication is a process language. We need a process language to help us navigate through life because we are human beings – growing and changing all the time. To begin to capture the fluidity of feelings and changes on a moment-to-moment basis and to communicate about our inner world, we need a process language. To be able to understand and accept other people for who they really are, including our clients, we need to have tools that open up communication so others feel safe revealing their true selves. Nonviolent communication gives us tools for speaking and listening in a new and powerful way.

The four steps in the process of Nonviolent Communication are:

- **Observation**
- **Feelings**
- **Needs**
- **Requests**

In the coming chapters, we'll work through each of these four steps in more detail, with opportunities to practice along the way.

CHAPTER 3

Step 1: Observation

The first step in NVC is Observation. NVC helps us shift our attention from labeling someone's actions or words as "right" or "wrong" (evaluation) to noticing what's going on in ourselves – and at the same time, really noticing or hearing what's going on in others (observation). This change in focus helps us become conscious of the important distinction between evaluation and observation.

TEASING APART OBSERVATION AND EVALUATION

Most of us blend our evaluations and observations together, so it can be difficult to separate the two. Learning to tease apart the difference, though, is a vital skill in Nonviolent Communication. An observation is akin to what a video or sound recorder can pick up; that is, it's a factual depiction of what happens, rather than an interpretive description of it. An evaluation, on the other hand, is our impression of an actual event. Evaluations can be judgments, labels, diagnoses, analyses, or speculations.

Example 1: The following story offers an example of how observations and evaluations can blur together:

Sandy had been seeing Lucy every Thursday for the last three months. Every time Lucy came to the office, she cried while talking about her life. Sandy tried to help her by advising and offering community resources that would provide more support for Lucy so she wouldn't feel so alone. No matter what she suggested though, Lucy continued to cry. Sandy felt frustrated and didn't know what she could do to help Lucy. "She's such a sad sack," Sandy thought.

At what point did Sandy's observation cross over into an evaluation? Did you notice that when Sandy began to feel frustrated she expressed her own frustration in the form of a label or an evaluation. "She's such a sad sack," is an analysis, a label, and an evaluation of what Lucy is. The evaluation says more about Sandy than it does about Lucy. The observation is that Lucy cries when she comes into the office. People continue to act a certain way until they get what they want. Lucy was not getting what she wanted from Sandy, so she continued to cry. Instead of Sandy's owning up to the difficulty she was having with Lucy, she used her position as a therapist to label and analyze Lucy. This can be very destructive if a client believes the labels placed on them by the expert. For instance, if Lucy takes on the label of "sad sack," she may live up to this identity by crying a lot. Labels, analysis, or other forms of static language will not take people to a place of healing. They will just muddy the water, creating more distress and confusion.

Example 2: Here's another example of the important distinction between observation and evaluation. This one comes from Sandy's journey:

When Sandy was asked "What is your client doing that bothers you?" she answered, "He's abusive and disrespectful."

Do the words "abusive" or "disrespectful" express an observation or an evaluation? _Hint_: A video camera cannot pick up someone being "abusive." It can pick up someone using cuss words though.

To change the evaluation "abusive" into an observation, Sandy might say: "He says, 'You fucking bitch.'" Though most of us can imagine the sting of those words, the observation statement itself is not emotionally charged. It is a neutral reporting of the observable facts of the situation. Those are, simply, the words that were spoken.

> Being able to adopt a neutral "observer stance" is an incredibly important skill for clinicians to practice.

Being able to adopt this neutral observer stance is incredibly important for therapists – it can help you detach from your emotional reactivity and give you a more powerful platform from which to communicate.

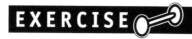

EXERCISE 3: PRACTICE OBSERVING

Think of someone who does not behave in a way that you like. Write down your observations of his or her behavior:

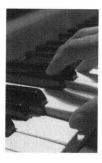

Now, look back at what you wrote and circle the observations you made. What behavior are you clearly observing? _HINT:_ Is the answer you wrote something a video camera can pick up?

Next, check: does your answer contain any evaluations? Underline any words you think seem evaluative. Remember, evaluations can be judgments, labels, diagnoses, analyses, or speculations – anything that adds a layer of meaning on top of the facts of the observed behavior.

CHAPTER 4

Step 2: Feelings

The second step of NVC is Feelings, and there are three important understandings about feelings that underlie the NVC process.

THREE KEY IDEAS ABOUT FEELINGS

First, from the perspective of NVC, feelings are neither good nor bad. They are just information about our internal world, information that can be observed without evaluation. When we have positive feelings, we know that our needs are being met. When we have negative feelings, we know that our needs are not being met.

> ### Three Important Ideas about Feelings
>
> 1. Feelings are neither good nor bad.
>
> 2. Feelings are not caused by other people.
>
> 3. Feelings teach you what your needs are and where you can work on healing.

Second, feelings are not caused by other people. This can be a tough one to get your mind around at first, because many of us are so accustomed to identifying the source of our feelings in others. "She made me so mad!" "He makes me happy." "Why do you have to worry me so?" From the NVC perspective, feelings may be triggered by others, but they are caused by something inside of us: our own needs.

Let's revisit Sandy to see how these first two ideas about feelings can play out. When Sandy's client cussed at her, she felt scared – not because of what he said, but because her need for safety and consideration was not met. The way Sandy feels about Bill and the needs she has in relation to him (and not what Bill says) determine how she feels. Even though Sandy is a professional, she still has feelings toward her clients because she is human. If she had no feelings, she would be dead.

Third, our own strong feeling responses teach us what our needs are and where we have inner work to do. In other words, our feelings are clues that lead us straight to those places in ourselves that are wounded and vulnerable. Taking responsibility for your own feelings means, in part, that you can begin to study what triggers strong feelings in you in order to learn where you are not healed. The more healed you are, the less you will be triggered by things other people say.

Your feelings also give you information about your needs. In the example, Sandy's feeling of fear told her that her needs for safety and consideration were not being met.

When you look back at these three key ideas about feelings, you may see that they add up to a strong model of personal emotional responsibility (which, interestingly, is also a model of personal freedom). When you believe the opposite of these three beliefs (that feelings can be judged as correct or shameful; that other people cause your feelings; and that you have no responsibility to learn from your feeling responses), you live in a frightening world in which you are always a potential victim.

When you believe that your feelings should be judged and that they are caused by others, you also perpetuate your own frustration and depression. How? Well, when you blame others for causing your negative feelings, that blame stimulates defensive reactions in others, and when people are preoccupied with defending against blame, they cannot (and don't particularly want to) meet your needs. In other words, when you express your needs in the form of blame, you are guaranteeing that those needs will not get met. And, when your needs are not met, you become depressed. Once you can take responsibility for your own feelings, you can live in a freer, happier, and more compassionate way.

PERSONAL ⊘ REFLECTION

REFLECTION TOPIC 3: NEW IDEAS ABOUT FEELINGS

What are your reactions to these ideas about feelings? Are these ideas different from how you've thought about feelings in the past? How so?

WHAT DO FEELINGS SOUND LIKE?

Take a look at some words we use to describe feelings. Isn't it amazing the rich vocabulary of feelings available to us? As you become more expert in using the language of feeling, you'll be able to convey nuances of experience that may surprise you! Notice that I've grouped them here not in terms of "good" or "bad" feelings, but rather in terms of the relationship between the feeling and the degree to which our needs are being met. Again, this is because in NVC, we move away from the notion that feelings are to be judged and toward the idea that feelings are clues to be learned from. (Consult the book, *Nonviolent Communication* by Marshall Rosenberg, for a more comprehensive feeling list.)

Words That Express Feelings When Needs Are Met

- affectionate
- loving
- tender
- absorbed
- engrossed
- fascinated
- involved
- hopeful
- optimistic
- open
- secure
- animated
- astonished
- energetic
- invigorated
- surprised
- appreciative
- touched
- wonder

- compassionate
- open hearted
- warm
- alert
- enchanted
- interested
- spellbound
- expectant
- confident
- proud
- excited
- ardent
- dazzled
- enthusiastic
- lively
- vibrant
- moved
- inspired
- joyful

- friendly
- sympathetic
- engaged
- curious
- entranced
- intrigued
- stimulated
- encouraged
- empowered
- safe
- amazed
- aroused
- eager
- giddy
- passionate
- grateful
- thankful
- awed
- amused

- delighted
- glad
- happy
- jubilant
- pleased
- tickled
- exhilarated
- blissful
- ecstatic
- elated
- enthralled
- exuberant
- radiant
- rapturous
- thrilled
- peaceful
- calm
- comfortable
- clear headed
- centered
- content
- equanimous
- fulfilled
- mellow
- quiet
- relaxed
- relieved
- satisfied
- serene
- still
- tranquil
- trusting
- refreshed
- enlivened
- rejuvenated
- renewed
- rested
- restored
- revived

Words That Express Feelings When Needs Are Not Met

- afraid
- apprehensive
- dread
- foreboding
- frightened
- mistrustful
- panicked
- petrified
- scared
- suspicious
- terrified
- wary
- worried
- annoyed
- aggravated
- dismayed
- disgruntled
- displeased
- exasperated
- frustrated
- impatient
- irritated
- irked
- angry
- enraged
- furious
- incensed
- indignant
- irate
- livid
- outraged
- resentful
- aversion
- animosity
- appalled
- contempt
- disgusted
- dislike
- hate
- horrified
- hostile
- confused
- ambivalent
- baffled
- bewildered
- dazed
- hesitant
- lost
- mystified
- perplexed
- puzzled
- torn
- disconnected
- alienated
- aloof
- apathetic
- bored

- cold
- distracted
- removed
- disquiet
- discombobulated
- perturbed
- shocked
- troubled
- uncomfortable
- unsettled
- embarrassed
- guilty
- fatigue
- depleted
- listless
- weary
- agony
- devastated
- hurt
- regretful

- detached
- indifferent
- uninterested
- agitated
- disconcerted
- rattled
- startled
- turbulent
- uneasy
- upset
- ashamed
- mortified
- beat
- exhausted
- sleepy
- worn out
- anguished
- grief
- lonely
- remorseful

- distant
- numb
- withdrawn
- alarmed
- disturbed
- restless
- surprised
- turmoil
- unnerved
- chagrined
- flustered
- self-conscious
- burnt out
- lethargic
- tired
- pain
- bereaved
- heartbroken
- miserable
- sad

- depressed
- dejected
- despair
- despondent
- disappointed
- discouraged
- disheartened
- forlorn
- gloomy
- heavy hearted
- hopeless
- melancholy
- unhappy
- wretched
- tense
- anxious
- cranky
- distressed
- distraught
- edgy
- fidgety
- frazzled
- irritable
- jittery
- nervous
- overwhelmed
- restless
- stressed out
- vulnerable
- fragile
- guarded
- helpless
- insecure
- leery
- reserved
- sensitive
- shaky
- yearning
- envious
- jealous
- longing
- nostalgic
- pining
- wistful
- repulsed

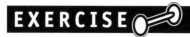

EXERCISE 4: NAMING YOUR FEELINGS

Using the above feeling words, imagine yourself in the following situation and write what you might be feeling:

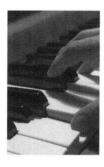

Your supervisor just told you that your client attempted suicide.

Someone is throwing stones at your window.

Your client says, "I don't want to work with you anymore."

You receive a card from your client's parents expressing their appreciation to you.

You are a single parent with two jobs and a young child.

You watch fireworks.

Your client says, "You listen with your head but not your heart."

Your boss says, "You are the brightest clinician in the company."

———————————————————————————

FEELINGS MIXED WITH EVALUATIONS

Some words sound like feeling words, but they are really evaluations of what other people are doing to you. Look at the list below and see if you can find where the evaluation comes in. Remember, evaluation is adding a layer of judgment or meaning on top of an observable feeling. An evaluation can also be defined as an observation mixed together with how you feel about it. NVC separates language, thereby making it more clear. A few of these words are:

Words That Express Evaluation or Judgment

- abandoned
- abused
- attacked
- betrayed
- cheated
- ignored
- interrupted

- let down
- manipulated
- misunderstood
- neglected
- patronized
- provoked

- put down
- rejected
- threatened
- unappreciated
- unwanted
- used

After taking some time to reflect on these words, look back at your responses to Exercise 4: Did you use any of these evaluative words? If you did, go back and see if you can change them to one of the feeling words from the lists of "Words that Express Feelings." This careful examination of the feeling words you use most often is a crucial step in the process of coming to take responsibility for your feelings. As you notice the language you habitually use, you will begin to catch yourself when you fall into language that implies blame or judgment of others, the language that keeps you stuck in a dependent position in relationships.

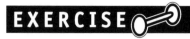

EXERCISE 5: WHAT DOES SELF-RESPONSIBILITY SOUND LIKE?

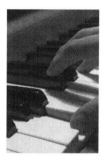 Take a look at the three statements in the table below. For each one, check the Yes or No box to indicate whether you think the speaker is expressing responsibility for his/her feelings:

	Taking Responsibility?	
	Yes	No
1. June says, "You hurt me when you say that."		
2. Myrna says, "I am irritated when I see your bike in the driveway because I would like to trust that our agreements will be kept."		
3. Jim says "You disappointed me when you stopped taking your medications."		

Check Yourself:

1. In this statement, June is naming the other person as the cause of her hurt. This is not expressing self-responsibility.

2. Myrna's feeling "irritated," is tied to her need, "trust." This is self-responsible.

3. Like June, Jim is claiming that the source of his disappointment is the person who stopped taking his or her medications.

How did you do? Are you getting the hang of what self-responsibility sounds like? Don't worry if you're not there yet – you'll have many more opportunities to practice.

REFINING HOW YOU SPEAK FROM FEELINGS

To review, the first level of learning to speak from feelings is to name a feeling, not an evaluation. The second level is to check whether you habitually shift from feeling statements to thought statements.

The purpose of NVC is to create heart connections with people. Sometimes we think we are expressing feelings, but we are really expressing thoughts. Expressing thoughts does not create heart connections. When expressing feelings, you can use this model: I feel_____. Fill in the blank with a feeling. Sounds easy, huh? Look at the list below and you'll begin to see how often we sidestep naming our feeling and instead voice a thought or an abstraction.

If you follow "I feel" with any of these words, you are probably expressing a thought, rather than a feeling:

- Like
- That
- As if
- As though
- I
- You
- He
- She
- It
- They
- Nouns or proper names

Here's an Example:

I feel like I did something wrong. This is a thought.

If it were a feeling, it would sound like this: *I feel ashamed because I think I did something wrong.*

I feel Henry should know better. This is a thought.

The thought statement could be changed to a feeling by saying: *When Henry admits to using cocaine, I feel scared because I want him to be safe.*

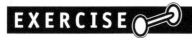

EXERCISE 6: REFINING YOUR STATEMENTS OF FEELING

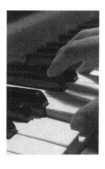 To begin this exercise, think of a time in your past when someone said something to you that triggered a strong reaction.

First, write down as best you can remember, what did that person say?

Now, put your feeling response into words: ***When s/he said that, I felt...***

When you are finished writing, look back at what you've learned about statements of feeling – did you really name feelings, not thoughts? Did you take responsibility for those feelings? GREAT! Can you find places in your language that suggest your feelings were caused by another person? What would it take to shift your language away from judgment and blame and toward self-responsibility for your feelings?

PERSONAL ⊘ REFLECTION

REFLECTION TOPIC 4: THE CHALLENGE OF SELF-RESPONSIBILITY

This chapter calls for changes in how you think about feelings and how you express feelings. For many of us, these can seem like BIG changes to make! As you look back at what you've learned about feelings in this chapter, which changes do you think will be most challenging for you to make? What changes do you most want to practice in the coming weeks?

CHAPTER 5

Step 3: Needs

The third step of Nonviolent Communication is to learn to identify needs – your own and others'. All human beings have needs, and many of those needs are universal; the core human needs are the same across cultures and time periods.

WHY NEEDS?

Needs are at the nucleus of each person. When we shift our attention from judging people to understanding what needs they are trying to meet by behaving in a certain way, we open up a safe space for dialogue. We also demonstrate understanding for what makes us human.

Communicating on the level of needs is deeply satisfying and creates such understanding between people that judgments dissolve. Being honest about our own needs allows others to see our humanness and makes it much easier to get our needs met. When we communicate our needs in terms of judgments, labels, analyses, or any of the other forms of habitual communication, it creates defensive reactions in others, and they don't want to give us what we are asking for.

SEVEN BASIC HUMAN NEEDS

There are seven basic classes of needs, according to NVC pioneer Marshall Rosenberg. These are:

- Autonomy
- Play
- Celebration
- Spiritual Communion
- Integrity
- Physical Nurturance
- Interdependence

The following list of needs is neither exhaustive nor definitive. It is meant as a starting place to support anyone who wishes to engage in a process of deepening self-discovery and to facilitate greater understanding and connection between people.

CONNECTION
acceptance
affection
appreciation
belonging
cooperation
communication
closeness
community
companionship
compassion
consideration
consistency
empathy
inclusion

intimacy
love
mutuality
nurturing
respect/self-respect
safety
security
stability
support
to know and be known
to see and be seen
to understand and
be understood
trust
warmth

**PHYSICAL
WELL-BEING**
air
food
movement/exercise
rest/sleep
sexual expression
safety
shelter
touch
water

HONESTY	AUTONOMY	efficacy
authenticity	choice	effectiveness
integrity	freedom	growth
presence	independence	hope
	space	learning
PLAY	spontaneity	mourning
joy		participation
humor	**MEANING**	purpose
	awareness	self-expression
PEACE	celebration of life	stimulation
beauty	challenge	to matter
communion	clarity	understanding
ease	competence	
equality	consciousness	
harmony	contribution	
inspiration	creativity	
order	discovery	

The contents of this page can be downloaded and copied by anyone so long as they credit CNVC as follows:

(c) 2005 by Center for Nonviolent Communication
Website: **www.cnvc.org** Email: **cnvc@cnvc.org** Phone: +1.505-244-4041

THE DIFFERENCE BETWEEN NEEDS AND STRATEGIES

Many of us in our culture are a bit confused about what our needs really are. For example, people in this culture often think that they need money. Is this really true? Remembering that core needs are universal, one quick way to check if something is a need is to ask yourself whether a person in a tribal culture needs it. Does the tribal person need money? The tribal person does not need money, but does need security and safety. Money is not a need. It is a strategy to meet a need.

it is important to differentiate needs from strategies
s are the human condition. Using communication to
he human being is very powerful. Once you under-
nen you will be able to create thousands of strategies
need. However, if you try to devise strategies before
understanding what need you are addressing, the strategy will probably not be effective in meeting the need.

EMPATHY: A UNIVERSAL NEED

Look back at the list of needs on page 55. Some of these words for
needs may seem confusing to you because they are not widely used in
our culture, such as the need for empathy. We all need empathy, but
we are not aware of this because we have rarely if ever experienced
it. Until we experience what it feels like to be received empathically,
we don't know what we are missing. Many therapists think they are
being empathic when they are really analyzing or educating. Using
empathy with your clients will open up the door to deeper explora-
tion because it creates safety. Empathy is such a crucial element of
NVC that we'll explore it in much greater detail in Chapters 7 and
8. For now, let's just look at what might happen if you began to empathize with your own needs.

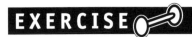

EXERCISE 7: EMPATHIZING WITH YOUR OWN NEEDS

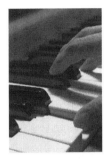

Let's look again at the list of universal needs:

Food, shelter, touch, safety, beauty, peace, celebration, empathy, honesty, love, reassurance, respect, support, trust, acceptance, connection, community, authenticity, creativity, and meaning

As you read each one, think about ways that need is met, or not met, in your life. Do any pop out of the list as being particularly lacking in your life?

Did you notice that "celebration" is a universal need? When was the last time you really celebrated? By celebrating day-to-day events when they occur or even before you go to bed at night, you will begin to notice the richness of the world, and your mood will respond positively. Keeping an appreciation journal is one way to begin this celebration process. Using NVC to write down what happened to you (observation), how you felt about it (feeling), and what need was met (need) will give you practice using NVC and will allow you to savor the experience. You can give yourself flowers or find a beautiful rock to remind you of what you are celebrating as you go through your day. As you look at the other needs, take a few minuets with each one to let yourself notice what feelings arise when you imagine each one of these needs being met. For instance when I think of my need for safety being met, I feel warm inside. When I think of the need for honesty being met, I feel excited because I value connection and growth. When people are honest, I have hope that these needs can get met.

Capture and write down your thoughts on where you are today in terms of your needs. As you go through this exercise, remember to do your best to suspend judgment about your needs. You are not being asked to say whether you think you deserve to have these needs or whether they are good or bad needs to have. Your goal is to reflect on what your needs actually are and the degree to which they are currently met or not met.

PERSONAL REFLECTION

REFLECTION TOPIC 5: NAMING YOUR NEEDS

How does it feel to you to name and think about your needs? What kinds of things can make it difficult for you to acknowledge your own needs?

AUTONOMY

Another need that is worth a closer look is the need for autonomy. Autonomy, *the need to be able to do and choose for yourself*, is a very strong need. For a quick image of what autonomy needs are, just picture a two-year-old. When you say "go," your two-year-old says "stop." When you say "please," your two-year-old says "no." "No" is the toddler's favorite word and a clear expression of the universal need for autonomy. When the expression of the need for autonomy is not received with compassion and understanding, it can go into hiding. Although hidden from our conscious awareness, the need can be triggered and expressed in ways that are destructive.

Autonomy needs can be triggered when a person hears or uses words like: should, shouldn't, have to, must, and ought. Words such as these create rebellion inside people – we react against the premise that we are subject to outside forces and not able to choose our own course of action. Think of how you might react if someone told you that you should change your hairstyle or that you ought to organize your sock drawer differently: you might find yourself thinking "Make me!" or "Since when are you the boss of me?" or "Who died and made you the dictator?" When you use these words when speaking to yourself, you may find yourself resisting doing something. For example when you think, "I have to get up now or I'll be late for work," you may find yourself rolling over and going back to sleep. Using this language internally or hearing it externally will create resistance. As you become more adept at using NVC, you will find that it's helpful to

> Autonomy needs can be triggered when a person hears or uses the words: *should, shouldn't, have to, must,* and *ought to.*

translate the shoulds, have to's and musts into feelings and needs. Instead of saying, "I have to get up now or I'll be late for work," you can say, "I'm feeling scared that if I don't get out of bed right now, I will be late for work for the third time this month and I could be fired. Since I don't have a different strategy to meet my need for security, I choose to get out of bed now." Noticing that we have the power to choose what we do moves us in the direction of self-responsibility. Instead of reacting to what others tell us we should do, we can hear the feelings and needs behind their "should" and decide whether or not we want to do as they suggest.

Sometimes when our autonomy needs are triggered, we may agree to do what someone is demanding of us but then assert our autonomy by not following through with that agreement. Have you ever wondered why patients don't do what they agreed to do? They are probably meeting their need for autonomy.

Are you requesting or demanding?

Often people are expressing autonomy needs when they don't carry out their promise to do something. Autonomy needs are triggered when people hear a demand. If you ask for something and punish the person if he/she doesn't do it, then you are making a demand and not a request. People sense a demand even when it is said nicely, using please. For instance, a nurse says to a patient, "Please don't use cocaine this week." This statement alone will not tell you if she is making a request or a demand. If you, the patient, use cocaine and at your next appointment she becomes angry and threatens to report you or threatens to quit being your nurse or threatens to admit you to a rehab center, then you know that she made a demand. If, however, you use cocaine and she empathizes with you, then you know she made a request. Demands imply punishment. In the face of demands most people either submit or rebel. When people submit, they loose their self-respect; when they rebel, they lose opportunities for connection. Both choices involve a reaction instead of a choice. An empowered person makes choices. Empowered people are conscious of their choice and act from a centered place inside of themselves when choosing instead of a place of reactivity. If you want to encourage cooperation, become conscious of whether you are making a demand or a request.

Think of the last time one of your requests was refused. How did you respond?

If you responded by calling names, giving the person the "silent treatment," or withholding something the person likes, then your request was actually a demand. If you were able to empathize with what prevented that person from meeting your request, then you probably made a request and not a demand.

NEEDS ARE LINKED TO FEELINGS

As we discussed in the section on feelings, unmet needs cause unpleasant feelings. Depression, frustration, anger, all are feeling responses – and important clues – to the fact that one or more of our needs are not being met. For instance, if our need for meaning is not fulfilled, we can trudge through our days going to work, taking care of the kids, or numbing out in front of the TV, but inside we will feel empty and tired.

Sometimes, we respond to this sense of emptiness by judging our-selves: *"I should get it together," "I'm just being lazy," "I need to try harder."*

Or we blame others: *"If my supervisor would allow me to work evening shift, then I would get to work on time"*... or, *"If they didn't give me so many clients, I'd perform better."*

Or we can respond by looking for escape by overeating, oversleeping, casting about for what might "fix" the bad feelings.

Or we can ask: *"What is this feeling teaching me? What need do I have that is not being met?"* and *"How can I begin to meet that need?"*

NVC suggests that the latter approach is more effective.

Once we understand what our needs are, we can figure out strategies to meet them. No longer will we waste our time and energy in un-conscious ways trying to meet our unconscious needs.

REFLECTION TOPIC 6: TAKING CHARGE OF YOUR NEEDS

The section above suggests that self-judgment, blame, and escape are common ways of avoiding taking responsibility for your own needs. When you think about shifting into the "driver's seat" and taking responsibility for getting your needs met, what do you think that would look like in your life? What kinds of actions could you take? (You might kick off your reflection by completing this sentence... "If I knew I were in charge of getting my own needs met, I would...")

HOW DO I KNOW WHAT MY NEEDS ARE?

If you are someone who is unused to naming and claiming your needs, you may find it quite challenging to describe to yourself – let alone to someone else – what you need. The good news is that there are some tricks you can use to help you discover those needs you've been unconscious of. One way to connect with our own needs is to think about what you don't want, and one way to discover that is to pay attention to what you are most judgmental about in others. Turns out, the very things that bug you most in others are the clues to what you need!

For instance, if I say:

"That person is totally insensitive."..
I need sensitivity.

"What a motor-mouth! She talks too much."..
I need to be heard.

"He is so patronizing, I hate it when he
treats me like I don't know anything."..
I need respect.

People often find it uncomfortable to express their needs directly. If you are scared of how others might react to the direct expression of your need, you will find the lesson on self-empathy helpful. If it is scary to hear "no" when you ask for something, then the lesson from Chapter 8: "Finding the Yes Behind the No" may be helpful.

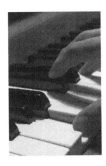

EXERCISE 8: UNCOVERING YOUR NEEDS

OK, now it's your turn! Try this exercise to see if you can uncover some needs you may not be acknowledging. (You may want to refer to your lists of feelings and needs to remind you of the language available to you.)

Draw a table with four columns and 5 rows:

Step One: In column 1, list the five people in your world who irritate or annoy you the most.

Step Two: In the second column, capture things you've thought or said that express your judgment of each person.

Step Three: In the third column, write down the feeling that you associate with your interactions with that person.

Step Four: Now, turn it around. What is the need that each of your judgments and feelings are pointing to?

ASKING FOR WHAT YOU WANT

Even when we do know what our needs are, it can be difficult to express them directly, for a variety of reasons.

I Shouldn't Have Needs

Many of us have been taught to give up our needs and take care of others and have developed shame about having needs at all. Our needs have gone into hiding from our own consciousness. Some of us may have been taught that our needs are a burden to others. We never learned how to ask for what we wanted because we were told that we were selfish or weak when we did so.

I Shouldn't Have to Tell You My Needs

Others of us harbor a wish that our needs should be fulfilled magically, without our having to play any role in that fulfillment. Ever heard (or thought) this one? "If you loved me, you'd know what I need." A very destructive – yet very common – belief is that when people really care for us, they should automatically intuit our needs and give us what we want without us having to ask for it and without our even being aware of what we want.

It takes insight and practice to learn to express our needs directly.

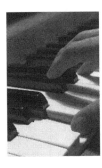
EXERCISE 9: DIRECTLY EXPRESSING YOUR NEEDS

Think of a time when you wanted something but were afraid to ask for it. Write down what you said or did in an attempt to get what you wanted:

Now write what you really needed, drawing from the list of Needs (page 42).

Have you ever been angry at or disappointed in someone for not meeting your needs? Did you expect that person to "just know" what your need was in the situation? Try "re-scripting" that experience: What would it sound like if you were to communicate your needs in words?

JUST ASK

In a nutshell, the answer to how to get your needs met is: ASK. Easier said than done, right? Learning to ask for what you want takes practice and requires a certain leap of faith. Interestingly, this leap will become easier and easier the more you practice asking for what you want. The more you ask for what you want, the more you will believe and understand that your needs are gifts to others. You may need to practice a lot of self-empathy, too, if you are scared to ask for what you want.

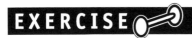
EXERCISE 10: PRACTICE ASKING

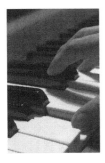

Think of something that is hard for you to ask for and write it down.

When you think of asking for this, how do you feel?

What is your feeling teaching you about your needs?

Here's Sandy's response to this same exercise (notice that if Sandy were to express her needs, it would benefit her and Bill):

"It is hard for me to ask my boss to schedule Bill with a different clinician. I'm scared he will think that I am a bad therapist and can't handle people who have schizophrenia. I want to be seen as competent so that my need for financial security will be met. I know that I am not helping Bill now because I am reactive to him. I imagine he might benefit more from working with someone else."

As you practice putting your needs into language, you'll begin to do better and better at actually getting those needs met. And as you get your needs met more often, you'll have fewer negative emotions and more stamina and energy to bring to the work of caring for others. As you may know, too many caregivers become burnt out because they don't take care of their own needs.

PERSONAL REFLECTION

REFLECTION TOPIC 7: WHEN IT WORKS TO ASK

Think back to a time when you successfully asked for what you needed. Some things you might want to recall include: What inner work did you do before you made the request? Did you get the response you expected? How did it work out?

CHAPTER 6

Step 4: Requests

The fourth step of Nonviolent Communication is the request. Becoming conscious about what we want back from another person when we express our feelings and needs directly is essential in creating connections and in building the life of our choosing. Communication is an act of creation. By being clear about what our needs are and by making clear requests of others, we can create a life that serves us in positive ways and that meets our needs to contribute to others.

Whenever we speak with other people, we want something back from them (otherwise we would be just as happy speaking to a wall). Becoming conscious of what you want back from people and what action they can take that would meet your needs is not easy. Our lack of clarity in this area can create confusion and stimulate hurt feelings.

For example, if you reflect on your objective in talking to someone, you may discover that your objective is to get the other person to change, or to get your own way. If this is the case, then your objective will inevitably defeat your attempt to develop a connection. People want to know that you care as much for their needs as you care for you own before they will be willing to drop their defenses and trust you.

If, on the other hand, your objective is to understand and to be understood, you'll be well-positioned to stay connected to the person with whom you are speaking. One way to accomplish your desire to be understood is to make clear requests using positive action language.

POSITIVE ACTION LANGUAGE

To make a clear request, ask for what you DO want, not for what you don't want. This is called using Positive Action Language. Here's an example of how Positive Action Language differs from other ways of making requests.

Sandy told her intern, "I don't want you wearing blue jeans to the office." The intern came in the next day wearing leggings and a tight shirt. Sandy realized she had not made a clear request. When making a clear request it is important to ask for what you *do* want, not for what you *don't*. Using the tools of NVC Sandy tried again to communicate with her intern. She said, "When I see you come to the office wearing certain clothes, I feel worried that your needs for respect won't be met and then I'll have to deal with the aftermath. Would you sit down with me for a few minutes and talk to me about what kind of image we want to project in this office and what kind of clothes will help that to happen?"

This kind of communication is much more likely to create the kind of unity and ease that Sandy is looking for. For one thing, when

Sandy failed to express her feelings and needs in the first request, the intern very likely heard her request as a demand. It is important to express our feelings and needs so others will understand where we are coming from and they are more likely to have compassion for us.

This is because human beings connect on the need level. All people have the same needs. It is easier to have compassion for someone with whom we can relate. It is also important to include others in decisions that affect them, since people are typically more willing to do something when they feel it is their decision.

There are two types of requests: connecting requests and action requests.

CONNECTING REQUESTS

When we begin to open up communication with others (especially after we have been speaking to them in our habitual fashion for years), it helps to make connecting requests. Connecting requests help to create connections between people so that it is possible for all to get their needs met. A connection is made when each person can accurately understand what feelings and needs are being expressed by the other. Creative solutions to problems can be created once the connection between people is established. Answers flow from this connection because by talking on this level, needs are clarified.

> Connecting Requests
>
> 1. "Can you tell me what you are hearing me say?"
>
> 2. "How do you feel when you hear me say this?"

1. Checking for Understanding

The first connecting request is: "Can you tell me what you are hearing me say?"

This simple question is a wonderful way to gauge if the person you are speaking with understands you accurately. It may take several attempts to be heard accurately. If the other person does not understand what you said, thank him/her for trying and repeat your message. The other person may be so blocked as to be unable to hear you after several attempts. In order to unblock that person, you may need to empathize with what is going on that prevents him/her from hearing you (refer to the section on empathy).

EXERCISE 11: MAKING A CONNECTING REQUEST

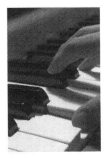

Think of a situation in which you are not being heard accurately. Write down how you would use the first connecting request (Can you tell me what you're hearing me say?) using the four steps of NVC:

Observation:

Feeling:

Need:

Request:

Sandy's response:

Observation: When I hear you say, "Fuck you"

Feeling: I feel scared

Need: Because my needs for safety and respect are not being met

Request: Can you tell me what you are hearing me say?

2. Checking for Feeling Responses

The second type of connecting request is a request for information about the feelings your message may trigger in the person with whom you are speaking. It sounds like this: "How do you feel when you hear me say this?"

Being open to hearing about the other person's feelings will allow us to know how our words are being received, what is being triggered, and what we next need to do to create a connection. As you listen to the feelings the other person is articulating, be very conscious that you did not cause those feelings, though you may have triggered them. Remember, those feelings are clues to the other person's unmet needs. Stay focused on uncovering those needs rather than getting sidetracked by guilt or worry that you have caused bad feelings.

ACTION REQUESTS

The second type of request is the action request. Action requests need to be doable in the present moment. An example of an action request might be: "Would you tell me if you would be willing to take the trash out every Tuesday?" Although the actual taking out of the trash will not occur until the next Tuesday, you are asking for an agreement in the present moment.

> An action request asks for a clear action that is doable in the present moment.

Action requests seem pretty straight forward, right? So how come people don't always follow through on what they've agreed to do?

When yes doesn't mean yes: the origins of resentment

Have you ever agreed to do something that was asked of you and then not followed through on that agreement? Is it possible that your lack of action could be traced back to saying "yes" when the real answer was "no"?

People say yes when they mean no for lots of reasons, but the effects of mixing up your yes's and no's are quite serious. When we forget how to say "no," then our "yes's" aren't reliable. Some people say yes because they are placing demands on themselves to please everyone and so they hear everything as a demand (the outer world reflects the inner world). Even if they do what you ask, they will probably feel resentment about it.

Resentment occurs when we do anything out of fear, shame, guilt, or obligation. This is one reason why it is important for us to find out how people feel about our requests. (And why it is so important to check with yourself as to how you are feeling about what others request of you!) To keep the relationship clear of resentment, we only want people to do something for us because it gives them pleasure to do it.

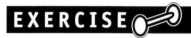

EXERCISE 12: REWINDING FROM RESENTMENT

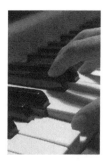 Think back to a time you felt resentful about something you were asked to do. Then, rewind in your mind to the moment when you agreed to do it. Was your "yes" a genuine yes? Or, were you acting out of fear, shame, guilt, or obligation? In the space below, rewrite your remembered scene – this time being truthful about your yes or no. How would it have sounded to say no? What might have happened next? What would have had to be different in the situation for you to have felt pleasure in taking the action that was requested of you?

PERSONAL ⊘ REFLECTION

REFLECTION TOPIC 8: REFLECTING ON THE FOUR STEPS

At first, expressing yourself using these four steps of the NVC process may be quite uncomfortable. Because it is so different from our habitual patterns, it does not feel normal. As you begin to try out the four steps: observation, feeling, need, request – how does it feel for you? What are some of the good things you are experiencing as you begin to practice with these tools in your life?

CHAPTER 7

Practicing Self-Empathy

HALFWAY THERE

Using the four steps of NVC you've just learned about – observations, feelings, needs, and requests – to express your honesty is the first step toward becoming a skilled compassionate communicator. The next big step in the process of NVC is to learn how to give empathy to others and yourself. Communication consists of speaking and listening. Nonviolent communication consists of speaking honestly and listening with empathy. It is empathy that allows you to take risks in communicating differently. In this chapter, we'll look closely at how you can begin to offer empathy to yourself, and in the next chapter, we'll focus in on how to extend empathy outward to others – even when it is very difficult to do.

SELF-CONNECTION PAVES THE WAY

Being able to empathize with yourself is an invaluable tool when you are dealing with people who are difficult for you to be around.

Self-empathy will help you stay connected with your own life energy and will prevent you from saying things that you will regret later. Self-empathy is a diverse tool that you can use anytime, anywhere, with anyone. It is about connecting with your own feelings and needs and by doing so, becoming more compassionate with yourself. When you realize that you are expressing a need every time you do or say anything, then you can begin to tune into your inner world and find out more about who you are.

MOVING AWAY FROM WORDS THAT WOUND

Some of the words that we are socialized to use can create violent reactions in ourselves and others. Some of these words are: *should, shouldn't, have to, must, suppose to, deserve.* When you are holding tight to a belief based on any of these words, chances are you feel pretty angry – remember that autonomy need we talked about in Chapter 5? – and when you feel angry, you are likely to be disconnected from your needs. To reconnect with yourself when you've been using these words requires a conscious effort to discover the real need underlying your anger. Below is a formula you can follow to dig below your anger to unearth your unmet needs.

Words that wound

"I should"
"I shouldn't"
"I have to"
"I must"
"I'm supposed to"
"I deserve"

SELF-EMPATHY: A FORMULA

1. Listen to what is going on in your head. Enjoy noticing the judgments, labels, "should thinking" that is going on. Sandy's example: *"When my client called me a bitch, I felt angry because I was thinking that he shouldn't speak to me that way. I thought that he was a hopeless case."*

> **A Formula for Self-Empathy**
>
> 1. Observe your thoughts without judgment.
>
> 2. Identify your unmet need(s).
>
> 3. Connect with how you feel about that unmet need.
>
> 4. Discover if there are other needs present you haven't considered?
>
> 5. Make a request for change.

2. Determine which need of yours is not met. Sandy's example: *"My needs for respect and safety were not met."*

3. Now connect with what feeling is alive in you when you determine your unmet need. Sandy's example: *"I feel scared."*

4. Check and see if other needs are now present that you weren't in touch with before. Sandy's example: *"I need to grow and learn new skills so I know how to deal with clients like Bill."*

5. Do you have a request to make to yourself or to the other person?

Sandy's example: *"The request I'll make to myself is to try to understand what's going on with me and with Bill when he speaks to me like that. I want to develop new communication skills so I can better take care of myself when faced with difficult clients."*

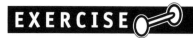
EXERCISE

EXERCISE 13: EXTENDING EMPATHY TO YOUR OWN ANGER

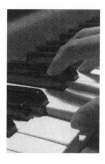

Now that you've seen how Sandy's situation fits into the formula, it's your turn to practice using it in your own life.

Step 1. Start by thinking of a time when you felt really angry. Describe the situation in one or two sentences: *A time I felt really angry was...*

Step 2. Now think back to that situation and write down what you remember about the thoughts you were having. (Remember, you are simply observing and recording these thoughts as if they are appearing on a tickertape in your mind. You are not judging or analyzing them – just reporting.) *The thoughts that were running through my head at that time were...*

Step 3. What were you needing? (Remember your lists of needs from Chapter 2? If you have trouble naming your needs, refer to that list.) *What I really needed was...*

Step 4. Now what do you feel? *When I think of those needs going unmet, I feel...*

Step 5. Check to see if there are any new needs surfacing? *To be honest, I also needed...*

Step 6: What request do you want to make of yourself or others? *I would like to request that...*

WHEN TO USE SELF-EMPATHY

When you find yourself in judgment

Self-empathy is especially useful when you are triggered by something that someone says or when you feel negative emotions that others may not know how to empathize with. A nurse who works on an inpatient psychiatric unit tells the following story about self-empathy:

"There was a patient on the unit who weighed 650 pounds. Every time he spoke to me I felt irritated. Instead of expressing the judgments and analysis that popped into my head, I shut my mouth and gave myself empathy and said nothing to this patient. After two days of doing this, the patient said to me, "You're the nicest nurse here." I was surprised to hear this because I had barely spoken to this patient. Then I reasoned that other people were probably equally triggered when he spoke, but instead of going inside for self-empathy, they expressed their judgments to the patient."

When you find yourself judging someone, begin by giving yourself empathy before attempting to empathize with her. If you are judging her and try to give her empathy anyway, it will sound like you are patronizing her. People can sense the energy behind our words. If the energy is not compassionate, then people distrust our empathy.

When you are pleased and happy

It can also be helpful to empathize with yourself when you are having positive feelings. Positive emotions are usually easier for others to empathize with, but it is important that you learn to empathize with all of your feelings – both unpleasant, pleasant and neutral. When you are in touch with your inner world of feelings and needs, then you are more likely to be in a centered place. When you are in a centered place, you'll be in a position to choose how you want to react to a situation. Instead of reacting habitually, you can choose to react to others in a way that is congruent with your spiritual values.

When you regret something that has happened in the past.

It is human to do things sometimes that you later regret. None of us is perfect! But, when you find that you are weighed down by regrets about your past, it can be very freeing to extend empathy towards yourself – or, more precisely, to the self you were back then. The exercise below can help you take the first step:

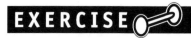
EXERCISE 14: EXPLORING THE NEEDS BENEATH YOUR REGRETS

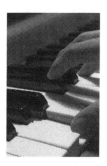

Think of a time when you did something that you regret. Write down what you did:

What need(s) were you trying to meet when you did this thing?

What needs did you not meet when you did this thing?

Here's what Sandy answered to these same questions:

"When my son was six, I went back to graduate school for two years. I spent those years studying and going to classes. I barely had time to see my son. I realize that I chose that strategy because I was scared of being able to make a living. I was meeting my need for security. However, I grieve the loss of connection with my son and the fact that I was not able to support him and meet his needs during that time. I failed to live up to my own values around parenting. Perhaps if I knew then what I know now, I could have figured out a different strategy that would have met both of our needs better."

PERSONAL REFLECTION

REFLECTION TOPIC 9: EXPERIENCING SELF-EMPATHY

As you begin to work on extending empathy toward yourself, what do you find most challenging? Is there a particular step in the "self-empathy" formula that you find to be a sticking point for you? Take a moment to share your experience with this self-empathy process.

CHAPTER 8

Practicing Empathy for Others

EMPATHETIC PRESENCE

Practicing empathy for others begins with self-empathy and also with the practice of empathetic presence. Self-empathy paves the way for empathetic presence by helping you get to a place where you can respond freely, unencumbered by judgments or anger.

Empathetic presence is not easy. It requires that we shed all judgments and preconceived ideas about a person and listen with our whole being, not merely with our ears. Most of us believe that we are empathic people, yet often the language we use to express our empathy sounds judgmental or analytical. When we advise, console, educate, interrogate, sympathize, analyze, explain, or correct, we are not empathizing. Empathy requires being present in the moment and open to the process that is unfolding.

Presence is not just an abstract concept; it is a tangible energy between people. Have you ever been in the middle of a conversation with a friend and suddenly realized that the friend was not fully present? How did you know? People can sense the quality of one another's presence, and they can definitely sense when that presence has drifted away. Even though your friend may still have been saying "uh huh," you could tell that he was not really there with you.

And what happens to you when you sense that the person you are communicating with is no longer present? You begin to shut down, interpreting that lack of presence as lack of interest or disrespect. Conversely, presence creates a sense of freedom and allows people to touch deeper levels of themselves.

EMPATHETIC LISTENING

When you are fully present, you can listen empathetically to what someone is saying. But how is empathetic listening different from other forms of listening? Below you'll see examples of how empathetic listening differs from some other common habits of response we saw first in Chapter 2.

The Initial Statement:

Sandy's client says, *"You're treating me like a little baby."*

Common Responses:

Analysis: "Your problem is that you are emotionally immature."

Active listening: "Sounds like you're upset about the way that I speak to you."

Advising: "If you would only take your medications, then you would feel better.

Correcting: "I am not treating you like a baby; I'm trying to help you."

Consoling: "I know that you are upset, but you'll feel better soon."

Educating: "The medication will help clear up your thinking."

Empathizing: **"Are you feeling frustrated and need to be treated with respect?"**

When someone is upset, anything we say can escalate the situation. Can you see that empathy is the least likely to create a defensive reaction? One way to see the difference is to look back at each of the responses and ask yourself what Sandy's client might say next. While the other responses invite an argument or a defensive reaction, the empathizing words are likely to trigger a response like "Yes, that's exactly how I feel" or "No, how I really feel is…" Either way, a connection has been made at the level that matters most to Sandy's client.

EXERCISE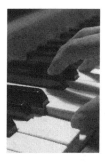

EXERCISE 15: FORMULATING EMPATHETIC QUESTIONS

Try formulating empathetic responses to the following statements. As you do, remember that it doesn't matter if you are exactly right about the person's feelings and needs – what matters is that you make an honest inquiry into them. What is the person feeling and needing when making the statements below?

Statement 1. "You never listen when I talk to you."
Write down what an empathetic response might be:

Statement 2: "You have ruined my life!"
An empathetic response might be: ...

Statement 3: "I wish I'd never been born."
An empathetic response might be: ...

Statement 4: "I never do anything right."
An empathetic response might be: ...

THE "FEELINGS AND NEEDS" MODEL OF EMPATHETIC RESPONSE

As we saw in the last exercise, when we empathize with people, we make an honest inquiry into what they are feeling and needing. We reflect back to them what we hear them expressing and ask whether our guesses about their feelings and needs are accurate.

It doesn't matter if our guesses are not accurate, because we can trust that if we are wrong, the person will tell us. So it doesn't matter if our guesses are right or wrong; what matters is that the process of guessing and being corrected will help us get closer to the truth of what the other person is trying to communicate.

To have empathy for someone is to clearly understand what feelings and needs are being expressed (either verbally or nonverbally) and to have compassion for the person expressing them. Having compassion can be tricky, however, when the person who is speaking to you expresses his need for empathy in the form of judgments, labels, or blame. In fact, the need for empathy is sometimes expressed in distorted ways that make it very difficult to see. For instance, a teenager who killed his parents said he did so because he just wanted them to understand what he felt like. His need was for empathy (understanding). The way he tried to get his need met (by killing his parents) did not get him the understanding that he was seeking; in fact it got him the opposite, judgment and punishment.

When you are working to empathize with someone who is judging you, blaming you, or lashing out at you, it can take real work to recognize what the feelings and needs are underneath what is being said. The payoff for doing this kind of work, though, is tremendous. If you can hear feelings and needs instead of thoughts and blame, then you will find that you don't take things personally even when they are directed at you. Wouldn't it be nice to be "immune" to blame and judgment?

Hearing distressed clients with heartfelt empathy will go a long way toward soothing them.

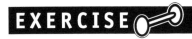

EXERCISE 16: HEARING THE NEEDS BENEATH THE JUDGMENT

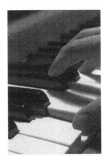
Here's a quick practice at listening for the feelings and needs below the surface of a critical, blaming statement.

Sandy's client, Bill, says: *"You fucking bitch, you don't give a damn."*

What is he feeling? _____

What does he need? _____

Sandy translated that sentence like this: *"Are you feeling angry and hurt because you need reassurance that you are cared for?"*

IMPORTANT NOTE ON BOUNDARIES: Notice that in Sandy's translation, she did not take responsibility for Bill's feelings. She connected his feelings to his unmet needs. She said: "Are YOU feeling... because YOU need... " If she took responsibility for causing his feelings she would have said: Are **you** feeling angry and hurt because **I** canceled our last appointment? Sandy remembered that she is not the cause of her client's feelings, so she took herself out of her language. By understanding that Bill's feelings are caused by his needs and not by her actions, Sandy can keep the boundaries clear between them. If she said, "Are YOU feeling angry because *I* canceled our last appointment?" she would have confused the boundaries. It is important that clinicians keep their boundaries clear in order to avoid burn out. Understanding how to use language can help you enjoy connecting with others without feeling responsible for their feelings.

WHEN EMPATHY IS DIFFICULT

Despite our best intentions and our genuine desire to empathize with others, all of us have moments when empathy is difficult to extend. These moments are important to notice and to work with, because – if we are willing to turn our attention inward – they can teach us

> The degree of empathy we have for ourselves is the degree that we are able to empathize with others.

about where we are stuck in ourselves. Being unable to empathize with someone is an indication that some issue or judgment we have is in the way. By focusing our attention inward toward our own feelings and needs, we can find out what is in the way of hearing others.

In order to be empathic toward others, we must first be clear and connected with ourselves. We can be present to others to the extent that we have done our own inner healing work. Using the tools of NVC, we can become clearer and more connected with ourselves and with others.

The dialogue below between Sandy and Bill was only possible after Sandy looked inward and worked with her own feelings and needs.

At first, Sandy said,

> "I don't know how to empathize with Bill's anger toward his parents. He's mad because they refuse to support him financially any longer. I have a lot of empathy for his parents but none for Bill. If I had a child who used drugs and stole my checkbook, writing checks and forging my name, I'd be furious, too, and would disown him."

After Sandy got some empathy for her own judgments and learned the NVC empathy tool she was able to offer the following empathy to Bill:

Bill: *"My stupid parents won't let me stay with them."*

Sandy: *"Are you feeling angry because you need support?"*

Bill: *"Yes, where are they when I need them?"*

Sandy: *"Do you feel hurt and need reassurance that you are cared for?"*

Bill: *"It's obvious they don't care, no one does."*

Sandy: *"Are you sad and lonely?"*

Bill: (crying) *"Yes, I've really fucked up my life."*

Sandy: *"Sounds like you feel regret and wish you had made different choices."*

Bill: *"I don't blame them for being mad after what I did to them. I wish they would give me another chance."*

Sandy: *"I hear that you are longing for connection with your parents.* (changing from an empathic question to a solution question) *Would you be interested in brainstorming ideas that might help you either reconnect with your parents or determine other ways to get your need for support met?"*

Sandy felt compassion toward Bill during this interview. When he took responsibility for what he had done, she felt relieved. Because of her verbal empathy, Bill felt safe enough to disclose what he was afraid he would be judged for. By understanding the positive intention or need people are meeting when they do something, it becomes safe for them to admit their deeper vulnerabilities. Instead of fighting and defending against judgments, people can be honest about their actions.

If you want someone to stop doing something, first empathize with the need he or she is meeting by engaging in the behavior you'd like to see changed. For example, if you want people to quit smoking, first empathize with the need they are meeting by smoking. (They may be meeting a need for belonging or connection or relaxation.) Once you can hear this without judgment, they may express their own concerns about what they are doing.

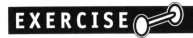
EXERCISE 17: WHEN EMPATHY IS DIFFICULT – START WITH YOURSELF

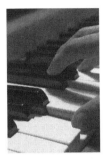

1. Begin this exercise by thinking about a time when you have real difficulty empathizing with a statement or message you received from your client. What did your client say that you had difficulty empathizing with?

2. Next, rather than trying to force an empathetic feeling that is not coming to you, step back and give yourself empathy for your own painful feelings and unmet needs.

When I hear this message, I feel...

This statement does not meet my needs for....

3. Once you've fully explored your own feelings and needs, go back and re-focus your attention on your client's statement. Now that you've acknowledged your own feelings and needs, can you begin to understand the feelings and needs that are being expressed by your client?

My best guess is that, when my client made that statement, he was feeling...

I think he probably needed...

USING EMPATHY TO UNBLOCK CONVERSATION

True communication is an art, a form of dance, in which two or more people alternate between speaking and listening. Knowing when to speak and when to listen will help you communicate more effectively – to truly hear and truly be heard. Often people cannot hear what you are saying because they need empathy. When that's the case, you may want to put whatever it is you want to say aside for a moment and "unblock" them by giving them the empathy they need. The dialogue below is an example of how such unblocking can occur.

Sandy (expressing her honest feelings and needs, and making a connection request):

"When you talk to me about your music being stolen from you, I feel confused because I want understanding for my perception of the situation. Can you tell me what you are hearing me say?"

Bill: *"You're wrong. My music did get stolen."* (Notice that he was unable to hear Sandy's message.)

Sandy: (empathizing) *"Are you feeling angry because you want acknowledgment for your point of view?"*

Bill: *"No one believes me."*

Sandy (Continuing to empathize): *"Are you lonely and need connection and a sense of belonging? You would like understanding for how painful it is for you when you think your music has been stolen. You feel scared that such a thing could happen and feel sad because you were hoping for the recognition that would come to you from your hard work."*

Bill: *"Yes, that's it."* (Bill may need hours of empathy before he can hear Sandy's message. The more pain people are carrying around, the less they will be able to hear until their pain is heard and understood.)

Sandy: *"I think I understand how it is for you. Now I'm wondering if you can listen to how it is for me. Would you be willing to do that now?"*

Bill: *"Okay."*

Sandy tries again to have her message received. By presenting her view of reality to Bill in such a compassionate manner, he is more likely to hear it, and it may help him begin to shift his old patterns and belief systems.

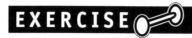

EXERCISE 18: WHEN YOUR HONESTY IS NOT GETTING THROUGH

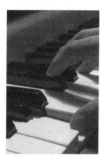

Think of a time when you expressed your honest feelings and needs. Write down what you said.

What response did you get back?

How did you feel when you heard this response?

Was your message received in the way you intended?

If not, imagine what feelings and needs were alive in the person who did not receive your message.

When you express your honesty, people may have reactions to what you share. Be ready to hear their feelings and needs even if what they say sounds like an attack. Until you are ready to receive whatever comes back, you may want to wait to disclose your honesty until you have support systems in place. You will feel safer trying these new tools if you know that you can get help with your own emotional reactions.

USING EMPATHY TO FIND THE "YES"

Remember reading in Chapter 5 that when people speak or act they are expressing a need? This holds true when someone says "no" to your request. If we can listen to what need they are expressing when they say "no," communication will open, allowing everyone's needs to get met. Hearing the Yes behind the No is also called Empathizing with the No.

Sandy (Expressing her honesty): *"When I notice how you are acting, I feel scared and need reassurance that you'll be safe. I'm wondering if you would be willing to sit down and talk with me so that we can work out a strategy that will give me the reassurance that I need."*

Bill: *"No, I don't want any part of your manipulation."*

Sandy (empathizing with the 'no'): *"Are you feeling tense and need reassurance that your needs matter as much as mine?"*

Bill: *"Well, they never have before."*

Sandy (Continuing to empathize): *"Do you distrust my intention and need reassurance that you won't be coerced into doing something you don't want to do."*

Bill: *"You've laid a power trip on me in the past, now I'm not doing anything you say."*

Sandy: *"Sounds like you need understanding for how that's been for you in the past and I'm also hearing that you have a need for autonomy, to make your own decisions about things."*

Bill: *"That's right; I'm a human being too.*

Sandy: *"Do you need to be treated with dignity and respect?"*

Bill: *"Yea, just like anyone else."*

Sandy: *"I understand why you might be reluctant to talk with me now, considering what happened in the past. I agree that I laid a power trip on you in the past because I was ignorant of how to get my needs met and also respect your needs. I would really like another chance now that I have learned a few things about communicating. Would you be willing to sit down and talk with me for twenty minutes so I can share some things I am learning with you?"*

As you can see, empathizing with the "no" opened up the dialogue and gave Sandy information about what was in the way of Bill's saying "yes." She learned that Bill needed empathy about how he was treated in the past and that he was holding onto pain and resentment about his needs not being respected. Now that she knows this, she can meet his needs for empathy and help create a caring connection between them. Out of this connection, Sandy and Bill can dialogue about how to get both their needs met and create win/ win solutions.

PERSONAL ⊘ REFLECTION

REFLECTION TOPIC 10: PRACTICING EMPATHETIC LISTENING

Find an occasion to practice empathetic listening. It can be almost any conversation – a conversation with a friend or family member will work fine. How did empathetic listening go for you? Did it change anything about the usual dynamic between you and the person with whom you were speaking?

QUESTIONS AND ANSWERS ABOUT EMPATHY

Q: How can I tell if my empathetic communication is working?

A: You know when someone has had enough empathy because they stop talking and there is a shift in their body language, or they breathe a big sigh.

Q: How do you empathize with someone who refuses to talk to you? Whenever I start to question my client, Molly, about her drug and alcohol use, she clams up and won't say anything.

A: There are several ways to empathize with a message like this. One way is to give Molly "silent empathy." This means silently understanding what feelings and needs she is expressing. Focusing your attention on her feelings and needs will help prevent you from taking it personally. It will help you be in a space to connect with her when she does start talking.

Another strategy is to give her empathy out loud. This may sound like, "Are you feeling scared and want to protect yourself from being judged and analyzed?" When she answers, reflect back what you are hearing her say.

A third strategy that can be used in this situation is to give yourself empathy. If you feel yourself react negatively when Molly does this, focus your attention on your own feelings and needs. This may sound like this: "I'm feeling nervous when she stops talking because I want to connect with what is going on with her. How can I help her if she won't talk to me?" Connecting with yourself first will soothe your feelings and may prevent you from saying something you regret.

Q: I hate it when a patient gets angry. How do I empathize with that?

A: First let's get clear about why you hate hearing your patient getting angry. Maybe it's because you think you need to do something to fix it, or you get scared. You can find this out by going inside and giving yourself empathy. Whenever we have a "negative" reaction to someone, it's an indication that we need empathy. After you give yourself empathy, focus your attention on your patient's feelings and needs. Empathy may sound like this: "Are you feeling angry and need understanding?" Continue to empathize as he gives you more information. Eventually he may stop expressing anger and sigh or say, "I feel better."

Q: How do I empathize with my clients when they talk about their delusional world?

A: Listen for the feelings and needs that they are expressing underneath their words. For example, when Bill said, "If you would only talk to me about how they stole my music, I'd be rich now" Sandy empathized with this by saying, "Are you feeling angry and need understanding?" By listening to the feelings and needs underneath the story, Sandy is helping Bill become reconnected to his own feelings and needs, and she is creating an emotional connection with him. This will help him trust her and will allow him to open up more.

CHAPTER 9
Conclusion

MY EXPERIENCE WITH NVC

As a trainer for the Center for Nonviolent Communication, I have had the opportunity to bring NVC to a wide array of audiences, and I am consistently impressed with the difference it can make in people's lives – from couples and parents to organizational leaders, NVC opens up new possibilities for everyone who works with it.

Parents who learn NVC experience a profound shift in their family dynamics. One parent said, "NVC saved my relationship with my children. Instead of raising my children the way I was raised, I was able to raise them in a loving way that was congruent with my inner values."

Couples who have divorced or separated will often learn how to connect with each other after learning NVC. I have seen many couples get back together after learning these tools. Whether or not couples get back together, they tell me their relationships become more harmonious and they are able to work out their differences. Nonviolent Communication is a powerful process for healing emotional pain and for developing self- empowerment. It dissolves blocks that prevent us from being all that we are.

NVC is also a powerful way to expand leadership skills. When I applied NVC to an international leadership test given by a large institution, I scored 98% - the highest score in the institution! In setting after setting, my experience has confirmed that the principles of NVC can lead to expansion of possibilities and profound change at every level: individual, organizational, and world.

I offer these tools here so that you can begin to apply them to becoming more empowered to create the relationships you'd like to have with your clients with mental illness. As you use these tools to become ever more congruent with who you are and what your values are, you can begin to be the change agent in your own life – transforming your ability to stay connected to others and yourself even through the most difficult of times. By using these tools in your work as therapist, you can begin to change the old paradigm of being the authority figure who has power over your clients to being a compassionate influence. Martin Buber, the philosopher, says true healing can only occur between equals where one heart is open to another. You can't force anyone to change, but you can make a profound contribution to their lives by offering compassion, empathy, and honesty.

NVC teaches that what we say to ourselves and to others creates the world we experience. When we become conscious of our communication and recognize that we can choose how we think and react, we change our world. My hope is that your world is improved with these tools. May you find ongoing support for that evolution.

FINDING SUPPORT FOR PRACTICING NVC

Nonviolent Communication practice groups are safe places to practice these new tools and get the empathy and support you need. The following web sites can give you more information about NVC and can connect you with local organizations: www.cnvc.org (international organization for the Center for Nonviolent Communication), www.nwcompass.org (local organization in Washington), www.dnadialogues.com (author's website)

PERSONAL REFLECTION

REFLECTION TOPIC 11: FEEDBACK ON THIS GUIDEBOOK

Reflecting back on your experience with this guidebook, please take a few minutes to share your comments: What about this guidebook was most helpful to you? Are there areas you would like to see expanded or issues you would like to read more about? Were there places you found confusing or unclear? Please let Melanie Sears know about your experience so that she can continue to enhance this book. www.dnadialogues.com

ABOUT THE AUTHOR
Melanie Sears

Melanie Sears has been a trainer for the Center of Nonviolent Communications since 1991. She trains businesses, hospitals, nursing homes, hospices, individuals, couples, and parents in the process of Nonviolent Communication and has presented Nonviolent Communication at conventions, at universities, and at churches. Her presentations have been described as exciting, inspiring, educational, and transformative, and she has helped to expand understanding about NVC through radio interviews, TV shows, articles, and other writings. Melanie says, "Everything is about communications. Any problem can be resolved within minutes when negative energy is transformed into caring connections."

In addition to her work with the Center for Nonviolent Communications, Melanie is an R.N. with over thirty years experience in all areas of the hospital, home care, and hospice. She has also been an administrator and a consultant. Her latest nursing position was as a psychiatric nurse on an acute inpatient unit. Her book, *Humanizing Health Care with Nonviolent Communication* describes her experience working on that unit, delves into the systems that make it difficult to receive compassionate care in the hospital, and illustrates how to apply Nonviolent Communication to create a more humane environment. She has two grown children and has just become a grandmother.

Other Publications by Author

Humanizing Health Care: Creating Cultures of Compassion with Nonviolent Communication by Melanie Sears

This intriguing, insightful book will give you a glimpse of horizontal violence among the staff and verbal violence toward patients that occur in our health care systems. With real examples, Sears takes you on a journey that will enlighten and inspire you. This is a must read for hospital administrators, health care workers and anyone who has been or will be a patient in a health care setting.

Puddle Dancer Press, Sept. 2010

Order it at www.nonviolentcommunication.com

Made in the USA
San Bernardino, CA
14 February 2016